The Growing Years: A Student's Journey into Pediatric Endocrinology

ORWELL

The Growing Years: A Student's Journey into Pediatric Endocrinology

Copyright © 2023 by ORWELL

The first edition was published in 2023

ISBN:
Published by:
Sunshine
1663 Liberty Drive
Hyderabad, IN 47403
www.Sunshinepublishers.com

This book is self-published using on-demand printing and publishing, which allows it to be printed and distributed globally

TABLE OF CONTENT

Chapter 4: Diagnostic Tools and Techniques in Pediatric Endocrinology 28

Physical Examination and Medical History Taking

Laboratory Tests for Hormone Assessment

Imaging Studies and Their Role in Diagnosis

Genetic Testing in Pediatric Endocrine Disorders

Chapter 5: Treatment and Management of Pediatric Endocrine Disorders 36

Medications and Hormone Replacement Therapy

Nutritional Management in Pediatric Endocrinology

Surgical Interventions for Endocrine Disorders

Psychological and Emotional Support for Patients and Families

Chapter 6: Multidisciplinary Approach in Pediatric Endocrinology 44

Collaboration with Pediatricians and Other Specialists

Role of Dieticians and Nutritionists in Treatment Plans

Psychologists and Social Workers in Pediatric Endocrinology

Chapter 10: Conclusion and Reflections on the Journey 69

Chapter 1: Introduction to Pediatric Endocrinology

Understanding the Field of Pediatric Endocrinology

Introduction:

Welcome to "The Growing Years: A Student's Journey into Pediatric Endocrinology." In this subchapter, we will explore the fascinating field of pediatric endocrinology, a branch of medicine that focuses on the study and treatment of hormonal disorders in children. Whether you are a medical student or simply curious about endocrinology, this chapter will provide you with a comprehensive understanding of the field.

What is Pediatric Endocrinology?

Pediatric endocrinology deals with the diagnosis and management of hormonal disorders in children, ranging from infancy to adolescence. These disorders can affect growth, puberty, metabolism, and overall development. By studying the intricate interplay between hormones and the body's various systems, pediatric endocrinologists help children lead healthier lives.

Common Conditions:

Pediatric endocrinology encompasses a wide range of conditions. Some common disorders include:

1. Diabetes: Type 1 and type 2 diabetes affect children of all ages. Understanding how to manage blood sugar levels and

provide appropriate insulin therapy is crucial for pediatric endocrinologists.

2. Growth Disorders: Conditions such as short stature or excessive growth can be caused by hormonal imbalances. Pediatric endocrinologists evaluate growth patterns and recommend appropriate interventions.

3. Puberty Disorders: Precocious puberty (early onset) or delayed puberty can significantly impact a child's physical and emotional development. Pediatric endocrinologists assess hormonal levels and provide appropriate treatments.

4. Thyroid Disorders: Conditions like hypothyroidism or hyperthyroidism can affect a child's metabolism, growth, and overall well-being. Pediatric endocrinologists monitor thyroid function and recommend appropriate medications.

5. Adrenal Disorders: Disorders such as congenital adrenal hyperplasia or adrenal insufficiency can affect hormone production, leading to various health issues. Pediatric endocrinologists diagnose these disorders and develop treatment plans.

Training and Expertise:

Becoming a pediatric endocrinologist requires years of specialized education and training. After completing medical school, aspiring doctors pursue a residency in pediatrics, followed by a fellowship in pediatric endocrinology. This comprehensive training equips them with the knowledge and skills to diagnose and manage hormonal disorders in children effectively.

Collaborative Approach:

Pediatric endocrinologists work closely with a multidisciplinary team, including nurses, dieticians, psychologists, and social workers. This collaborative approach ensures comprehensive care for children with hormonal disorders. They also collaborate with other specialists, such as surgeons or radiologists, when necessary.

Conclusion:

Understanding the field of pediatric endocrinology is crucial for medical students and individuals interested in endocrinology. By delving into the complexities of hormonal disorders in children, we can appreciate the importance of pediatric endocrinology in improving the lives of young patients. Whether you choose to specialize in this field or simply want to expand your knowledge, "The Growing Years" is your guide to unlocking the mysteries of pediatric endocrinology.

Importance of Pediatric Endocrinology in Children's Health

As students venturing into the field of endocrinology, it is essential to understand the significant role that pediatric endocrinology plays in the overall health and well-being of children. Pediatric endocrinology focuses on the diagnosis and treatment of hormone-related disorders in children, specifically those related to growth, development, and metabolism. This subchapter aims to shed light on the importance of pediatric endocrinology and its impact on children's health.

One of the primary reasons pediatric endocrinology is crucial is its role in identifying and addressing growth disorders in children. Growth is a vital aspect of a child's development, and any abnormalities in growth patterns can indicate an underlying endocrine disorder. Pediatric endocrinologists are trained to assess and treat conditions such as short stature, delayed or precocious puberty, and growth hormone deficiencies, ensuring that children receive appropriate interventions to optimize their growth potential.

Another significant area of concern is the impact of pediatric endocrine disorders on a child's metabolism. Hormones play a crucial role in regulating metabolism, and any disruptions can lead to conditions like diabetes, thyroid disorders, or obesity. Pediatric endocrinologists are equipped to diagnose and manage these conditions, providing children with the necessary tools and guidance to lead healthy lives.

Additionally, pediatric endocrinology is vital in addressing the emotional and psychological well-being of children. Hormonal imbalances, especially during puberty, can have profound effects on a child's mental health. Conditions such as gender dysphoria or disorders of sexual development require the expertise of pediatric endocrinologists who can provide comprehensive care and support to children and their families.

Furthermore, pediatric endocrinology plays a pivotal role in ensuring the long-term health of children with endocrine disorders. By closely monitoring hormone levels, managing medications, and providing ongoing support, pediatric endocrinologists help children navigate the challenges associated with chronic conditions, improving their quality of life and reducing the risk of complications.

In conclusion, pediatric endocrinology plays a crucial role in promoting children's health and well-being. By addressing growth disorders, metabolic conditions, emotional well-being, and long-term management, pediatric endocrinologists provide comprehensive care to children with endocrine disorders. As students exploring the field of endocrinology, it is essential to recognize the importance of pediatric endocrinology in shaping the lives of children and contribute to their optimal health outcomes.

Overview of Hormones and their Role in Growth and Development

Hormones play a crucial role in the growth and development of our bodies. They are chemical messengers that are produced by various glands in our endocrine system. These glands, such as the pituitary gland, thyroid gland, and adrenal glands, release hormones into the bloodstream, where they travel to different parts of the body to carry out their functions.

In this chapter, we will explore the fascinating world of hormones and understand how they influence our growth and development. Whether you are a student studying endocrinology or simply curious about the workings of your body, this knowledge will provide valuable insights into the complex processes that occur within us.

One of the key hormones involved in growth and development is the growth hormone (GH), which is produced by the pituitary gland. GH stimulates the bones and tissues to grow, ensuring that we reach our full height potential during adolescence. It also plays a role in maintaining healthy body composition and metabolism.

Another important hormone is insulin, which is produced by the pancreas. Insulin regulates blood sugar levels and allows glucose to enter cells, providing them with the energy they need to function. Any imbalance in insulin production can lead to conditions such as diabetes, affecting growth and development.

Additionally, thyroid hormones, produced by the thyroid gland, play a significant role in growth, brain development, and metabolism. These hormones are essential for maintaining the overall health of our bodies and ensuring proper development during childhood and adolescence.

The adrenal glands, situated on top of the kidneys, release hormones such as cortisol and adrenaline, which help us respond to stress and regulate our body's response to different situations. These hormones also contribute to the development of secondary sexual characteristics during puberty.

Throughout this chapter, we will delve deeper into the specific functions of these and other hormones, exploring their effects on various aspects of growth and development. We will also discuss common endocrine disorders that can arise when these hormones are not produced or regulated properly.

Understanding the role of hormones in growth and development is essential for anyone interested in endocrinology or studying the human body. By grasping the intricate connections between hormones and our physiological processes, we can gain insights into the mechanisms that shape our bodies and discover potential treatments for endocrine disorders.

Join us on this exciting journey into the world of pediatric endocrinology, as we uncover the mysteries of hormones and their impact on growth and development.

Chapter 2: Basics of Pediatric Endocrinology

Anatomy and Physiology of the Endocrine System

Welcome to "The Growing Years: A Student's Journey into Pediatric Endocrinology." In this subchapter, we will dive into the fascinating world of the anatomy and physiology of the endocrine system. As students interested in endocrinology, it is essential to comprehend the intricate workings of this system to better understand the field.

The endocrine system is a network of glands that secrete hormones directly into the bloodstream. These hormones act as chemical messengers, regulating various bodily functions and maintaining homeostasis. Understanding the anatomy of this system is crucial for identifying the glandular structures involved.

The major glands of the endocrine system include the hypothalamus, pituitary gland, thyroid gland, parathyroid glands, adrenal glands, pancreas, ovaries, and testes. Each gland plays a vital role in ensuring the body's overall health and development.

To grasp the physiology of the endocrine system, let's explore two important components: hormones and feedback mechanisms. Hormones are chemical substances produced by endocrine glands that travel through the bloodstream to target organs or tissues. They regulate growth, metabolism, reproduction, and many other bodily functions.

Feedback mechanisms are crucial in maintaining hormone balance. Negative feedback loops are the most common mechanism, wherein the body senses hormone levels and adjusts secretion accordingly. For instance, if blood glucose levels are high, the pancreas releases insulin to lower it. Once the glucose levels stabilize, insulin secretion decreases.

The endocrine system works in harmony with other body systems, notably the nervous system. The hypothalamus and pituitary gland form a vital link between the two. The hypothalamus produces releasing hormones that signal the pituitary gland to release or inhibit specific hormones. This interaction ensures coordination between the nervous and endocrine systems.

Understanding the anatomy and physiology of the endocrine system is the foundation for studying pediatric endocrinology. As students, it is essential to recognize the normal functioning of this system to identify and address any potential health concerns in children.

In summary, the endocrine system is a complex network of glands that produce hormones to regulate bodily functions. By understanding the anatomy and physiology of this system, you can delve deeper into the field of endocrinology and contribute to the well-being of children. Keep exploring and developing your knowledge in pediatric endocrinology to make a significant impact on the lives of young patients.

Hormone Regulation and Feedback Mechanisms

In the fascinating world of endocrinology, hormone regulation and feedback mechanisms play a vital role in maintaining the delicate balance of our body's functions. As students diving into the realm of pediatric endocrinology, it is crucial to understand how these processes work and their significance in our overall health and development.

Hormones are chemical messengers secreted by various glands in our body, including the pituitary gland, thyroid gland, adrenal glands, and many others. These hormones travel through our bloodstream, acting as signals to different organs and tissues, instructing them on how to function. The regulation of these hormones is essential for maintaining homeostasis, or the stable internal environment of our bodies.

One of the key components of hormone regulation is the negative feedback mechanism. This mechanism acts as a control system that maintains hormone levels within a specific range. When hormone levels rise above the desired range, the feedback mechanism signals the gland to reduce hormone secretion. On the other hand, if hormone levels fall below the desired range, the feedback mechanism stimulates the gland to increase hormone production. This delicate balance ensures that our body functions optimally.

Let's take an example to understand this better. The thyroid gland produces a hormone called thyroxine, which regulates metabolism, growth, and development. When thyroxine levels decrease, the hypothalamus, a region in our brain, releases thyrotropin-releasing hormone (TRH). TRH then signals the pituitary gland to release thyroid-stimulating hormone (TSH). TSH, in turn, stimulates the thyroid gland to produce and release more thyroxine, bringing its levels back to normal. Once the thyroxine levels are within the desired range, the negative feedback mechanism halts the release of TRH and TSH, ensuring balance.

Understanding hormone regulation and feedback mechanisms is crucial in diagnosing and treating endocrine disorders. Imbalances in hormone levels can lead to various conditions such as growth disorders, diabetes, and thyroid disorders. By studying these mechanisms, students can gain valuable insights into how these disorders occur and how to effectively manage them.

In conclusion, hormone regulation and feedback mechanisms are fundamental concepts in the field of endocrinology. As students venturing into pediatric endocrinology, it is essential to grasp these concepts to understand the intricate workings of our bodies. By comprehending the delicate balance maintained by these mechanisms, we can unlock the mysteries of endocrine disorders and contribute to the well-being of our patients.

Key Hormones in Pediatric Endocrinology

In the world of pediatric endocrinology, hormones play a crucial role in regulating various bodily functions and development processes. Understanding the key hormones involved is essential for students venturing into the field of endocrinology. In this subchapter, we will explore the fundamental hormones that are central to pediatric endocrinology.

1. Growth Hormone (GH): GH is one of the primary hormones responsible for normal growth and development in children. Produced by the pituitary gland, it stimulates the growth of bones, muscles, and organs. A deficiency in GH can lead to growth disorders such as short stature, while excess GH can result in gigantism or acromegaly.

2. Thyroid-stimulating Hormone (TSH): Produced by the pituitary gland, TSH stimulates the thyroid gland to produce thyroid hormones that are essential for metabolism, growth, and development. Abnormal levels of TSH can indicate thyroid dysfunction, including hypothyroidism or hyperthyroidism.

3. Insulin: Produced by the pancreas, insulin regulates glucose metabolism in the body. It allows cells to take in glucose from the bloodstream, providing energy for growth and development. Insufficient insulin production or resistance to its effects can lead to diabetes mellitus, a condition characterized by high blood sugar levels.

4. Cortisol: Produced by the adrenal glands, cortisol is involved in regulating metabolism, immune response, and stress. It plays a crucial role in maintaining blood pressure and glucose levels. Disorders related to abnormal cortisol levels include Cushing's syndrome (excess cortisol

production) and adrenal insufficiency (insufficient cortisol production).

5. Sex Hormones: Estrogen and testosterone are key sex hormones that play a vital role in sexual development, puberty, and reproduction. Estrogen is responsible for the development of secondary sexual characteristics in females, while testosterone is responsible for the same in males. Imbalances in sex hormone levels can lead to conditions such as precocious puberty or delayed puberty.

Understanding the roles and functions of these key hormones is crucial for students studying pediatric endocrinology. It forms the foundation for diagnosing and managing various endocrine disorders in children. By comprehending the intricacies of these hormones, students can contribute to the field of endocrinology and help improve the health and well-being of pediatric patients.

In the upcoming chapters, we will delve deeper into each hormone, exploring their regulation, pathways, associated disorders, and management strategies. By gaining a comprehensive understanding of these key hormones in pediatric endocrinology, students will be better equipped to provide optimal care for their future patients.

Chapter 3: Common Pediatric Endocrine Disorders

Growth Disorders: Causes and Management

In the fascinating world of pediatric endocrinology, one of the most intriguing aspects is the study of growth disorders. As students diving into this field, we embark on a journey to understand the causes and management strategies for these disorders. Growth disorders encompass a range of conditions that can impact a child's physical development, often leading to concerns and challenges for both the child and their caregivers.

Causes:
To comprehend growth disorders, it is crucial to explore their underlying causes. Understanding the intricate mechanisms of the endocrine system is fundamental. Hormones play a vital role in regulating growth, and any disruptions in their production or function can lead to growth disorders. Genetic factors, hormonal imbalances, nutritional deficiencies, and certain medical conditions can all contribute to these disorders. As students, we must delve into the intricacies of these causes to unravel the mysteries of growth disorders.

Management:
The management of growth disorders is a collaborative effort between pediatric endocrinologists, nutritionists, and other healthcare professionals. Identifying the specific cause of the disorder is the first step towards effective management. Hormone replacement therapy, nutritional interventions, and growth hormone treatments are some of the strategies employed to address these disorders.

However, it is crucial to consider the individual needs of each child and tailor the management plan accordingly.

A holistic approach is essential when managing growth disorders. Regular monitoring of growth parameters and hormone levels is necessary to assess the progress and make necessary adjustments to the treatment plan. Additionally, providing emotional support to the child and their family is vital, as growth disorders can have a significant impact on their psychosocial well-being.

As students in the field of endocrinology, we have the opportunity to contribute to the advancement of knowledge in growth disorders. Research plays a vital role in understanding the underlying mechanisms, identifying new treatment modalities, and improving the overall management of these conditions. By staying updated with the latest scientific advancements and contributing to the body of knowledge, we can make a significant impact in the lives of children affected by growth disorders.

In conclusion, growth disorders present an intriguing and challenging aspect of pediatric endocrinology. By exploring the causes and management strategies, we can develop a comprehensive understanding of these disorders. As students, we have the opportunity to contribute to the field, make a difference in the lives of affected children, and pave the way for future advancements in the management of growth disorders.

Diabetes Mellitus: Types, Symptoms, and Treatment

Diabetes Mellitus is a chronic medical condition that affects millions of people worldwide. In this subchapter, we will explore the different types of diabetes, their symptoms, and the available treatments. Understanding these aspects is crucial for students interested in the field of endocrinology, as diabetes is a prevalent condition in pediatric endocrinology.

Types of Diabetes Mellitus:

There are three main types of diabetes: type 1, type 2, and gestational diabetes. Type 1 diabetes, also known as juvenile diabetes, usually develops during childhood or adolescence when the immune system mistakenly attacks and destroys insulin-producing cells in the pancreas. Type 2 diabetes, on the other hand, is more common in adults and is often associated with poor lifestyle choices, such as an unhealthy diet and sedentary behavior. Gestational diabetes occurs during pregnancy and usually resolves after childbirth.

Symptoms of Diabetes Mellitus:

Common symptoms of diabetes include increased thirst and hunger, frequent urination, unexplained weight loss, fatigue, and blurred vision. Type 1 diabetes symptoms may develop rapidly, while type 2 diabetes symptoms may be more gradual and subtle. It is important to recognize these symptoms early on to prevent complications and seek appropriate medical care.

Treatment of Diabetes Mellitus:

The primary goal of diabetes treatment is to keep blood sugar levels within a target range to avoid long-term complications. Type 1 diabetes is managed through insulin injections or the use of an insulin pump, as the body no longer produces insulin. Type 2 diabetes treatment often involves lifestyle modifications, such as adopting a healthy diet, engaging in regular physical activity, and sometimes taking oral medications or insulin injections if necessary. Gestational diabetes is typically managed through diet and exercise, and in some cases, insulin may also be required.

In addition to medical treatment, diabetes management also includes regular blood sugar monitoring, education on carbohydrate counting, and awareness of potential complications. It is important for students interested in endocrinology to understand these treatment approaches to provide effective care and support to patients with diabetes.

In conclusion, diabetes mellitus is a complex condition with various types, symptoms, and treatment options. As students exploring the field of endocrinology, it is crucial to grasp the fundamentals of diabetes management to make a positive impact on the lives of individuals with diabetes. By understanding the types, symptoms, and treatment approaches, we can contribute to the field of pediatric endocrinology and help improve the lives of those affected by diabetes.

Thyroid Disorders: Hypothyroidism, Hyperthyroidism, and Congenital Hypothyroidism

Welcome to the subchapter on thyroid disorders! In this section, we will explore three common conditions related to the thyroid gland: hypothyroidism, hyperthyroidism, and congenital hypothyroidism. As students interested in endocrinology, understanding these disorders is crucial to gaining a comprehensive knowledge of pediatric endocrinology.

Firstly, let's delve into hypothyroidism. This condition occurs when the thyroid gland fails to produce enough thyroid hormone. Students often wonder what causes hypothyroidism. Well, it can be due to an autoimmune disease called Hashimoto's thyroiditis, in which the body's immune system mistakenly attacks the thyroid gland. Other causes include iodine deficiency, certain medications, and radiation therapy. Symptoms of hypothyroidism may include fatigue, weight gain, constipation, and even depression. It is essential to diagnose and manage hypothyroidism early to prevent complications such as stunted growth and intellectual disability.

On the other end of the spectrum is hyperthyroidism, which occurs when the thyroid gland produces an excessive amount of thyroid hormone. Graves' disease, an autoimmune disorder, is the most common cause of hyperthyroidism in children. Some symptoms of hyperthyroidism include weight loss, rapid heartbeat, irritability, and difficulty concentrating. Treatment options for hyperthyroidism may include medication, radioactive iodine therapy, or even surgery. Understanding the underlying causes and appropriate management of hyperthyroidism is crucial to ensure optimal growth and development in affected children.

Lastly, we will discuss congenital hypothyroidism, a condition present at birth where the thyroid gland is absent or not functioning properly. Early detection and treatment are vital for infants with this condition, as untreated congenital hypothyroidism can lead to severe intellectual and growth delays. Newborn screening programs are in place to identify affected infants promptly. Treatment involves lifelong thyroid hormone replacement therapy.

As students interested in endocrinology, gaining a comprehensive understanding of thyroid disorders is essential. Remember, the thyroid gland plays a vital role in regulating various bodily functions, including metabolism and growth. By familiarizing ourselves with the causes, symptoms, and management of hypothyroidism, hyperthyroidism, and congenital hypothyroidism, we can contribute to the field of pediatric endocrinology and make a difference in the lives of children affected by these disorders.

In conclusion, this subchapter has provided an overview of three common thyroid disorders: hypothyroidism, hyperthyroidism, and congenital hypothyroidism. By studying these conditions, students interested in endocrinology can gain valuable insights into the diagnosis, management, and treatment options available for children with thyroid disorders. Remember, the thyroid gland is a vital component of the endocrine system, and understanding its disorders is crucial for providing optimal care to our young patients.

Disorders of Puberty: Precocious Puberty and Delayed Puberty

Puberty is a significant milestone in every individual's life, marking the transition from childhood to adulthood. However, for some students, this natural process may not occur at the expected time or may happen too early, leading to disorders of puberty. In this subchapter, we will explore two common disorders of puberty: precocious puberty and delayed puberty.

Precocious puberty refers to the early onset of puberty, occurring before the age of 8 in girls and before the age of 9 in boys. This condition can have a profound impact on a student's physical and emotional development. Students experiencing precocious puberty may notice the development of secondary sexual characteristics, such as breast development in girls and enlargement of the testicles in boys, at a significantly younger age than their peers. This can lead to feelings of self-consciousness and confusion, as they may not be mentally prepared for these changes. It is crucial for students and their families to seek medical advice if they suspect precocious puberty to ensure appropriate management and support.

On the other hand, delayed puberty is characterized by the absence of secondary sexual characteristics by the age of 13 in girls and 14 in boys. This condition can be distressing for students as they may feel left behind their peers in terms of physical development. It is essential to understand that delayed puberty can have various causes, including hormonal imbalances, genetic factors, chronic illnesses, or malnutrition. Students experiencing delayed puberty should consult a healthcare professional who specializes in endocrinology to determine the underlying cause and receive appropriate treatment if necessary.

Both precocious puberty and delayed puberty require careful evaluation and management by pediatric endocrinologists. These specialists are trained to diagnose and treat hormonal disorders that affect growth and development in children and adolescents. They will conduct a thorough medical history, physical examination, and may order additional tests to determine the underlying cause of these disorders.

Understanding disorders of puberty is vital for students interested in endocrinology. By familiarizing themselves with these conditions, students can gain insights into the importance of hormonal regulation and its impact on growth and development. As future healthcare professionals, students can play a crucial role in educating their peers and raising awareness about these disorders to ensure timely diagnosis and appropriate management.

In conclusion, disorders of puberty, such as precocious puberty and delayed puberty, can significantly impact a student's physical and emotional well-being. By seeking medical advice and understanding the underlying causes, students can work towards managing these conditions effectively. Through increased awareness and education, students interested in endocrinology can make a positive difference in the lives of those affected by these disorders.

Chapter 4: Diagnostic Tools and Techniques in Pediatric Endocrinology

Physical Examination and Medical History Taking

In the field of pediatric endocrinology, physical examination and medical history taking are essential components of evaluating and diagnosing various endocrine disorders in children. This subchapter will provide students with a comprehensive understanding of the importance and techniques involved in these aspects of patient assessment.

The physical examination is a crucial step in the diagnostic process as it allows healthcare providers to observe and assess the physical characteristics and signs associated with endocrine disorders. Students will learn about the significance of a thorough examination, including the measurement of height, weight, and body mass index (BMI). They will also delve into the examination of growth patterns, pubertal development, and the assessment of secondary sexual characteristics. The subchapter will provide detailed explanations and guidelines on how to perform these examinations accurately and the significance of each observation.

Moreover, students will gain insights into the importance of medical history taking when evaluating endocrine disorders in children. They will learn about the specific questions to ask regarding the patient's growth, development, and any associated symptoms. Understanding the family history and potential genetic factors will also be emphasized. The subchapter will guide students through the process of obtaining a comprehensive medical history, ensuring they have the necessary knowledge and skills to effectively gather crucial information.

Furthermore, this subchapter will highlight the significance of effective communication and building rapport with pediatric patients and their families during the physical examination and medical history taking. Students will learn the art of creating a comfortable and safe environment for patients, ensuring they feel heard, understood, and involved in their healthcare journey. The subchapter will provide tips and techniques for effective communication, enabling students to develop strong patient-doctor relationships.

In conclusion, the physical examination and medical history taking play a vital role in the evaluation and diagnosis of endocrine disorders in children. This subchapter in "The Growing Years: A Student's Journey into Pediatric Endocrinology" will equip students with the necessary knowledge and skills to perform accurate physical examinations and gather comprehensive medical histories. By mastering these essential components, students will be well-prepared to embark on their journey into the fascinating field of pediatric endocrinology.

Laboratory Tests for Hormone Assessment

In the field of endocrinology, laboratory tests play a crucial role in assessing hormone levels and diagnosing various endocrine disorders. These tests help healthcare professionals gain insights into the functioning of the endocrine system and provide valuable information for accurate diagnosis and treatment. This subchapter will delve into the laboratory tests commonly used to evaluate hormone levels in pediatric endocrinology.

Blood tests are the most frequently used method for hormone assessment. Through a simple blood draw, various hormones can be measured accurately. For instance, thyroid-stimulating hormone (TSH) and free thyroxine (T4) levels help evaluate thyroid function, which is essential for growth and metabolism. Additionally, insulin-like growth factor 1 (IGF-1) and growth hormone (GH) tests aid in assessing growth disorders.

Another important laboratory test is the cortisol test, which measures cortisol levels in the blood or urine. Cortisol is a hormone secreted by the adrenal glands, and its levels can indicate adrenal insufficiency or excess, both of which can have significant effects on the body.

Urinary hormone testing is also employed in endocrinology. The 24-hour urine test helps evaluate hormone levels over a longer period, providing a more comprehensive view of hormone secretion patterns. This test is particularly useful in assessing conditions such as Cushing's syndrome or adrenal hyperplasia.

In some cases, specialized tests may be required to evaluate specific hormones. For instance, the follicle-stimulating hormone (FSH) and luteinizing hormone (LH) tests help assess puberty development and reproductive function. Insulin and glucose tests are used to diagnose and monitor diabetes. These specialized tests require more specific protocols and are typically performed in specialized laboratories.

It is important to note that laboratory tests are just one part of the diagnostic process. They are used in conjunction with clinical assessments, medical history, and physical examinations to form a comprehensive understanding of a patient's endocrine health.

Understanding laboratory tests for hormone assessment is crucial for students interested in pediatric endocrinology. By familiarizing themselves with these tests, students can develop a better understanding of hormone disorders and contribute to the field. Moreover, this knowledge allows students to interpret test results accurately and collaborate effectively with healthcare professionals in the diagnosis and treatment of pediatric endocrine disorders.

In conclusion, laboratory tests form an integral part of hormone assessment in pediatric endocrinology. Blood tests, urinary tests, and specialized tests help evaluate hormone levels and provide valuable insights into the functioning of the endocrine system. By understanding these tests, students can contribute to the field of endocrinology and aid in the accurate diagnosis and treatment of hormone disorders in children.

Imaging Studies and Their Role in Diagnosis

In the field of pediatric endocrinology, imaging studies play a crucial role in the diagnosis and management of various conditions. These non-invasive techniques provide valuable insights into the structure and function of organs and tissues, aiding healthcare professionals in making accurate diagnoses and determining appropriate treatment plans. In this subchapter, we will explore the different imaging studies commonly used in pediatric endocrinology and their significance in clinical practice.

Ultrasound is one of the most frequently employed imaging techniques in pediatric endocrinology. It uses high-frequency sound waves to create images of internal organs and is particularly useful in assessing the thyroid gland, adrenal glands, and reproductive organs. Ultrasound can help identify abnormalities such as nodules, cysts, or tumors, providing valuable information for diagnosis and guiding treatment decisions.

Another commonly used imaging study is magnetic resonance imaging (MRI). This technique uses a powerful magnetic field and radio waves to create detailed images of the body's internal structures. MRI is particularly valuable in evaluating pituitary gland abnormalities, such as tumors or cysts, which might cause hormonal imbalances. It can also help identify structural anomalies in the brain or spinal cord that may contribute to endocrine disorders.

Computed tomography (CT) scans are occasionally used in pediatric endocrinology when a more detailed evaluation of a specific area is required. CT scans provide cross-sectional images of the body, allowing for a comprehensive assessment of organs and tissues. They are particularly useful in identifying adrenal gland tumors or abnormalities in the pituitary gland.

Nuclear medicine imaging techniques, including positron emission tomography (PET) and single-photon emission computed tomography (SPECT), are employed in cases where functional information is required. These techniques involve injecting a small amount of radioactive material into the body, which is then detected by a specialized camera. PET and SPECT scans can help evaluate the functional status of various organs and tissues, aiding in the diagnosis and management of endocrine disorders.

In summary, imaging studies are indispensable tools in the field of pediatric endocrinology. Ultrasound, MRI, CT scans, and nuclear medicine techniques provide valuable information about the structure and function of organs, aiding in accurate diagnosis and treatment planning. As students in endocrinology, understanding the role of these imaging studies will enhance our ability to interpret and analyze patient data, ultimately improving our patient care and outcomes.

Genetic Testing in Pediatric Endocrine Disorders

Genetic testing is an essential tool in diagnosing and managing pediatric endocrine disorders. It helps healthcare professionals gain valuable insights into the underlying causes of these disorders, enabling them to provide more targeted and personalized care to patients. In this subchapter, we will explore the importance of genetic testing in pediatric endocrinology and its implications for patients.

Pediatric endocrine disorders are conditions that affect the hormone-producing glands in children and adolescents. These disorders can have a significant impact on growth, development, and overall health. While some endocrine disorders are caused by environmental factors or lifestyle choices, others have a genetic basis.

Genetic testing involves analyzing a patient's DNA to identify specific gene mutations or variations that may be contributing to their endocrine disorder. It can be done through various methods, such as blood tests, saliva samples, or even by examining a patient's skin cells. Once the genetic mutation is identified, healthcare professionals can better understand the underlying mechanism of the disorder and tailor treatment plans accordingly.

One of the key advantages of genetic testing in pediatric endocrine disorders is its ability to provide early and accurate diagnoses. By identifying the specific gene mutation responsible for a disorder, healthcare professionals can initiate treatment promptly, minimizing the potential complications associated with delayed diagnosis. Moreover, genetic testing can also help identify individuals who may be carriers of certain genetic conditions, allowing for proactive family planning and genetic counseling.

Additionally, genetic testing plays a crucial role in predicting disease progression and prognosis. By understanding the genetic makeup of patients, healthcare professionals can anticipate the potential complications or associated conditions that may arise later in life. This knowledge allows for better long-term management and monitoring of patients with pediatric endocrine disorders.

However, it is important to note that genetic testing in pediatric endocrine disorders is not without limitations. Some gene mutations may be rare or unique to an individual, making them challenging to detect using conventional testing methods. Furthermore, the interpretation of genetic test results requires expertise, as the significance of certain gene mutations may still be unknown or subject to ongoing research.

In conclusion, genetic testing is an invaluable tool in the field of pediatric endocrinology. It helps healthcare professionals in diagnosing and managing endocrine disorders, providing personalized and targeted care to patients. By understanding the genetic basis of these conditions, we can improve early diagnosis, predict disease progression, and optimize treatment plans. Genetic testing empowers both healthcare professionals and patients, enabling them to make informed decisions regarding their health and future.

Chapter 5: Treatment and Management of Pediatric Endocrine Disorders

Medications and Hormone Replacement Therapy

As students delving into the fascinating field of endocrinology, it is crucial to understand the role of medications and hormone replacement therapy in treating various endocrine disorders. Medications play a vital role in restoring hormonal balance and managing conditions that affect the endocrine system.

One of the most common uses of medications in endocrinology is hormone replacement therapy (HRT). HRT involves the administration of hormones to individuals whose bodies are unable to produce sufficient amounts naturally. This therapy is commonly prescribed for conditions such as hypothyroidism, growth hormone deficiency, and adrenal insufficiency.

For instance, individuals with hypothyroidism have an underactive thyroid gland, leading to decreased production of thyroid hormones. In such cases, synthetic thyroid hormones, such as levothyroxine, are prescribed to supplement the body's thyroid hormone levels. This medication helps patients regain energy, improve metabolism, and maintain a healthy weight.

Another condition that often requires HRT is growth hormone deficiency (GHD), which affects children and adults. For those with GHD, recombinant human growth hormone (rhGH) is prescribed to stimulate growth and development. This therapy can significantly enhance height, bone density, muscle mass, and overall quality of life in affected individuals.

Hormone replacement therapy is not limited to these conditions alone. It is also used to manage adrenal insufficiency, a condition where the adrenal glands fail to produce sufficient cortisol. In such cases, medications like hydrocortisone or prednisone are prescribed to replace the deficient cortisol and maintain adequate adrenal function.

Aside from HRT, medications are also employed to manage other endocrine disorders. Insulin, for example, is a vital medication for individuals with type 1 diabetes or type 2 diabetes who require insulin therapy. It helps regulate blood sugar levels and prevents complications associated with diabetes.

Furthermore, medications are used to manage conditions like hyperthyroidism, Cushing's syndrome, and polycystic ovary syndrome (PCOS). These medications aim to control the production of hormones, alleviate symptoms, and restore hormonal balance.

As students, understanding the role of medications and hormone replacement therapy is crucial in comprehending the management and treatment of various endocrine disorders. It is important to stay updated with the latest research and developments in this field to provide the best care and support to patients.

In conclusion, medications and hormone replacement therapy play a significant role in the field of endocrinology. They are indispensable tools in managing various endocrine disorders, restoring hormonal balance, and improving the quality of life for patients. Continual learning and staying abreast of advancements in this field will enable students to become knowledgeable and compassionate practitioners in the realm of pediatric endocrinology.

Nutritional Management in Pediatric Endocrinology

In the field of pediatric endocrinology, proper nutrition plays a significant role in the overall health and development of children. The growing years are a critical period for children, and it is during this time that their bodies require essential nutrients for optimal growth and hormonal balance. This subchapter explores the importance of nutritional management in pediatric endocrinology, providing students with a comprehensive understanding of how diet can impact the endocrine system.

The foundation of nutritional management in pediatric endocrinology lies in a balanced and varied diet. Students will learn about the different food groups and their specific importance in supporting the growth and development of children. Emphasis will be placed on the role of macronutrients such as carbohydrates, proteins, and fats, as well as micronutrients like vitamins and minerals. Students will explore how these nutrients contribute to the production and regulation of hormones in the body.

Furthermore, this subchapter will delve into specific nutritional considerations for children with endocrine disorders. Students will gain insight into how certain conditions, such as diabetes or thyroid dysfunction, can impact dietary requirements. They will learn about the importance of blood sugar regulation in diabetes management and how to calculate insulin doses based on carbohydrate intake. Additionally, students will understand the significance of iodine in thyroid disorders and the role of dietary modifications in managing these conditions.

To provide a practical understanding of nutritional management, case studies and real-life scenarios will be included throughout the subchapter. Students will have the opportunity to analyze and develop dietary plans for children with various endocrine disorders, applying their knowledge to real-world situations.

Furthermore, this subchapter will touch upon the role of nutrition education in promoting healthy habits among children and their families. Students will explore strategies for effectively communicating nutritional information to patients and their parents, emphasizing the importance of a collaborative approach to achieve optimal outcomes.

By the end of this subchapter, students will have a solid foundation in nutritional management in pediatric endocrinology. They will understand the significance of a balanced diet in supporting hormonal balance and growth in children. Armed with this knowledge, students will be well-equipped to provide comprehensive care to pediatric patients in the field of endocrinology.

Surgical Interventions for Endocrine Disorders

In the field of pediatric endocrinology, surgical interventions play a crucial role in the management of various endocrine disorders. While medical treatments are often the first line of defense, surgery becomes necessary in certain cases where other interventions have proven ineffective or when the condition is severe and requires immediate attention. In this subchapter, we will explore the different surgical interventions used to treat endocrine disorders in children.

One of the most commonly performed surgical procedures in pediatric endocrinology is thyroidectomy, which involves the removal of all or part of the thyroid gland. This procedure is typically recommended for children with thyroid cancer, goiter, or hyperthyroidism that does not respond to medication. Thyroidectomy may be performed using traditional open surgery or minimally invasive techniques such as laparoscopic or robotic-assisted surgery, which offer smaller incisions, reduced scarring, and faster recovery times.

Another surgical intervention is adrenalectomy, the removal of one or both adrenal glands. This procedure is indicated in cases of adrenal tumors or adrenal hyperplasia, conditions that can lead to hormone imbalances and other health complications. Adrenalectomy can be performed through open surgery or minimally invasive techniques, depending on the size and location of the tumor.

Pancreatectomy, the removal of all or part of the pancreas, is another surgical option for certain endocrine disorders such as insulinomas or pancreatic tumors. This procedure aims to eliminate the source of excessive hormone production and restore normal function to the pancreas.

However, due to the vital role of the pancreas in digestion and blood sugar control, this surgery is only considered when all other treatment options have been exhausted.

In addition to these specific surgeries, there are also general surgical interventions that may be required in the management of endocrine disorders. These include lymph node dissection, which is performed to remove cancerous lymph nodes in cases of metastatic disease, and organ transplantation, such as pancreas or adrenal gland transplantation, for patients with end-stage organ failure.

It is important for students in the field of endocrinology to have a good understanding of surgical interventions for endocrine disorders. While these procedures are not always the first choice, they can significantly improve the quality of life for children with severe or unresponsive conditions. By working closely with surgeons and other healthcare professionals, pediatric endocrinologists can determine the most appropriate course of action for their patients, ensuring the best possible outcomes.

Psychological and Emotional Support for Patients and Families

In the field of pediatric endocrinology, providing comprehensive care goes beyond just addressing physical health. It is equally important to offer psychological and emotional support to patients and their families. Dealing with endocrine disorders can be an overwhelming experience, especially for young patients and their loved ones. This subchapter will explore the significance of psychological and emotional support in pediatric endocrinology and how it can positively impact the overall well-being of patients and families.

From the moment of diagnosis, patients and their families often experience a range of emotions, including fear, confusion, and anxiety. As students entering the field of endocrinology, it is crucial to understand the psychological impact these conditions can have on individuals. By recognizing and empathizing with their emotional state, you can better support them throughout their journey.

Psychological support involves creating a safe and supportive environment for patients and their families to express their concerns and fears. Active listening, empathy, and open communication are essential skills in providing psychological support. By actively involving patients in their treatment plans and addressing any emotional barriers, you can enhance their overall experience and improve treatment outcomes.

Additionally, emotional support plays a vital role in pediatric endocrinology. Patients and families often face significant lifestyle changes, such as dietary modifications, medication management, and regular medical appointments. These adjustments can be challenging and may impact their emotional well-being. As students, it is crucial to assist patients and families in understanding and adapting to these changes while offering encouragement and motivation.

Furthermore, psychological and emotional support can extend beyond the patients themselves. Families of pediatric endocrinology patients also require support as they navigate the challenges and uncertainties that come with managing their child's condition. Providing resources, counseling services, and connecting families with support groups can be invaluable in helping them cope with the emotional toll of their child's diagnosis.

In conclusion, psychological and emotional support is an integral part of pediatric endocrinology. As students entering this field, understanding the importance of providing comprehensive care that addresses not only physical health but also psychological well-being is crucial. By implementing effective strategies for psychological and emotional support, you can contribute to improved patient outcomes and help families navigate the challenges they may face during their journey in pediatric endocrinology.

Chapter 6: Multidisciplinary Approach in Pediatric Endocrinology

Collaboration with Pediatricians and Other Specialists

One of the key aspects of pediatric endocrinology is the collaboration and teamwork between pediatricians and other specialists. As students venturing into the field of endocrinology, it is crucial to understand the importance of working together with different healthcare professionals to provide comprehensive care for young patients.

Pediatricians play a vital role in recognizing and managing endocrine disorders in children. They are often the first point of contact for families and are responsible for assessing the overall health and development of their patients. By collaborating with pediatricians, we can ensure accurate diagnosis and early intervention for endocrine conditions.

In the field of endocrinology, it is common to encounter complex cases that require the expertise of multiple specialists. It is essential to establish effective communication channels and foster interdisciplinary collaboration to provide the best possible care for children with endocrine disorders. Working alongside specialists such as radiologists, geneticists, surgeons, and nutritionists allows us to take a holistic approach to patient management.

Collaboration between pediatric endocrinologists and radiologists is particularly crucial in diagnosing and monitoring endocrine disorders. Radiologists play a vital role in interpreting imaging studies such as X-rays, ultrasounds, and MRIs, which aid in identifying structural abnormalities in hormone-producing organs. By working closely with radiologists, we can accurately interpret these images and guide appropriate treatment plans.

Geneticists also play a significant role in understanding the genetic basis of many endocrine disorders. Collaboration with genetic specialists helps us identify genetic mutations that may contribute to the development of endocrine conditions. This knowledge is crucial for personalized treatment plans and genetic counseling for families.

Surgical intervention may be necessary for certain endocrine conditions. Collaborating with pediatric surgeons allows us to discuss the surgical options available and ensure the best possible outcome for our patients. Additionally, nutritionists play a vital role in managing endocrine disorders that affect metabolism and require dietary modifications. Collaborating with them ensures that patients receive appropriate nutritional support.

In conclusion, collaboration with pediatricians and other specialists is essential in the field of pediatric endocrinology. By working together, we can provide comprehensive care, accurate diagnosis, and personalized treatment plans for children with endocrine disorders. As students embarking on a journey into pediatric endocrinology, it is vital to recognize the value of teamwork and interdisciplinary collaboration for the well-being of our young patients.

Role of Dieticians and Nutritionists in Treatment Plans

In the field of pediatric endocrinology, the role of dieticians and nutritionists in treatment plans is crucial. As students exploring the fascinating world of endocrinology, it is essential to understand the vital contribution these professionals make in improving the health and well-being of young patients.

Dieticians and nutritionists are experts in the study of food and its impact on the human body. They play a significant role in the treatment of children with endocrine disorders by developing personalized nutrition plans that support their overall health and address specific conditions. These professionals work closely with pediatric endocrinologists, nurses, and other healthcare providers to ensure comprehensive care for their patients.

One of the primary responsibilities of dieticians and nutritionists is to assess the nutritional needs of children with endocrine disorders. By considering factors such as age, weight, height, and underlying medical conditions, they develop customized meal plans that help optimize growth and development while managing the specific condition. For instance, children with diabetes may require a balanced diet that regulates blood sugar levels, while those with thyroid disorders may need foods rich in iodine and selenium.

Furthermore, dieticians and nutritionists educate patients and their families about the importance of a healthy diet in managing endocrine disorders. They provide valuable information on portion control, food choices, and the significance of nutrients like vitamins and minerals. By empowering families with knowledge, they enable them to make informed decisions about their child's nutrition, leading to improved treatment outcomes.

Collaboration with other healthcare professionals is a fundamental aspect of a dietician's and nutritionist's role. They work closely with pediatric endocrinologists to monitor the progress of patients and make necessary adjustments to the nutrition plan. This teamwork ensures a holistic approach to treatment and allows for timely interventions when needed.

In conclusion, dieticians and nutritionists play a vital role in the treatment of children with endocrine disorders. Their expertise in understanding the impact of food on the body, developing personalized nutrition plans, and educating patients and families is invaluable. By working collaboratively with pediatric endocrinologists and other healthcare providers, they contribute to the overall well-being and improved health outcomes of young patients. As students delving into the fascinating field of endocrinology, it is essential to recognize and appreciate the significant role dieticians and nutritionists play in the treatment plans of children with endocrine disorders.

Psychologists and Social Workers in Pediatric Endocrinology

As a student venturing into the field of pediatric endocrinology, it is crucial to understand that providing comprehensive care to young patients goes beyond medical treatment alone. In fact, a multidisciplinary approach is often required to address the complex needs of children and adolescents with endocrine disorders. This subchapter aims to shed light on the important roles of psychologists and social workers in pediatric endocrinology, highlighting their contributions and the unique perspective they bring to the table.

Psychologists play a vital role in supporting the mental and emotional well-being of young patients dealing with endocrine disorders. These professionals are trained to assess and intervene in areas such as anxiety, depression, body image concerns, and coping skills. By utilizing various therapeutic techniques, they help children navigate the challenges associated with their conditions, promoting resilience and improved quality of life.

In addition to psychological support, social workers are instrumental in addressing the social determinants of health that impact pediatric patients with endocrine disorders. They collaborate with families to identify and access necessary resources, including financial assistance, educational support, and community programs. Social workers also provide valuable guidance on transitioning from pediatric to adult healthcare, ensuring a seamless continuum of care as patients grow older.

The collaboration between psychologists, social workers, and pediatric endocrinologists is essential in facilitating holistic care. This multidisciplinary approach allows for a comprehensive understanding of patients' physical, emotional, and social needs, leading to improved outcomes and overall well-being.

One area where psychologists and social workers play a pivotal role is in the management of chronic conditions such as diabetes. With their expertise in behavior change and adherence, these professionals assist patients and families in developing effective self-care strategies. They also address the psychosocial impact of chronic illness, helping young individuals navigate the emotional challenges associated with their condition.

Furthermore, psychologists and social workers contribute to research and education within the field of pediatric endocrinology. They provide valuable insights into the psychological and social aspects of endocrine disorders, enriching our understanding and guiding the development of more effective interventions.

In conclusion, the inclusion of psychologists and social workers in pediatric endocrinology teams is essential for comprehensive and patient-centered care. Their expertise in mental health, social determinants of health, and behavior change greatly enhances the quality of life for children and adolescents with endocrine disorders. As students entering this field, it is crucial to recognize and embrace the collaborative nature of pediatric endocrinology, working hand in hand with these professionals to provide the best care possible for our young patients.

Chapter 7: Research and Advances in Pediatric Endocrinology

Current Studies and Clinical Trials in Pediatric Endocrinology

As students delving into the fascinating field of pediatric endocrinology, it is essential to stay up-to-date with the latest research and clinical trials. In this subchapter, we will explore some of the most exciting and promising studies happening in the field of pediatric endocrinology today.

1. Genetic Discoveries: Recent advancements in genetic research have shed light on the underlying causes of various endocrine disorders. Studies are underway to identify the specific genes responsible for conditions like growth hormone deficiency, congenital adrenal hyperplasia, and hypothyroidism. Understanding these genetic mechanisms will pave the way for more personalized treatments and interventions tailored to each patient's unique genetic makeup.

2. Growth Hormone Therapy Optimization: Growth hormone therapy has revolutionized the treatment of children with growth disorders. Ongoing studies aim to optimize the dosage and timing of growth hormone administration to maximize its effectiveness while minimizing side effects. Researchers are also investigating alternative modes of growth hormone delivery, such as long-acting formulations and transdermal patches, to improve patient adherence and convenience.

3. Diabetes Management Innovations: Diabetes is a prevalent endocrine disorder among children, and research is focused on improving its management. Clinical trials are

exploring novel insulin formulations, including ultra-rapid-acting insulins, to achieve better glucose control and reduce the risk of hypoglycemia. Additionally, researchers are investigating closed-loop systems, often referred to as artificial pancreas, which use algorithms to monitor blood glucose levels and automatically adjust insulin delivery.

4. Psychological Impact of Endocrine Disorders: The psychological well-being of children with endocrine disorders is a critical aspect of their overall health. Recent studies are examining the psychological impact of conditions like Turner syndrome, Klinefelter syndrome, and congenital adrenal hyperplasia. Researchers aim to develop interventions to promote mental health and provide support for these children and their families.

5. Long-Term Outcomes: Understanding the long-term effects of endocrine disorders and their treatments is crucial for optimizing patient care. Studies are tracking children with conditions like precocious puberty, congenital hypothyroidism, and type 1 diabetes into adulthood to assess their overall health, reproductive outcomes, and quality of life. This longitudinal research will provide valuable insights into the lifelong implications of pediatric endocrine disorders.

By keeping abreast of these current studies and clinical trials, students can contribute to the evolving field of pediatric endocrinology. As future endocrinologists, it is our responsibility to engage with research and strive for advancements that will enhance the lives of children with endocrine disorders. Remember, knowledge is power, and by staying informed, we can make a difference in the lives of our future patients.

Emerging Therapies and Technologies

In the dynamic field of pediatric endocrinology, advancements in therapies and technologies are constantly reshaping the way we approach and manage various conditions. These emerging treatments provide hope for better outcomes, improved quality of life, and enhanced patient care. As students diving into the world of endocrinology, it is crucial to stay updated on the latest breakthroughs and discoveries. This subchapter will delve into some of the most promising emerging therapies and technologies in pediatric endocrinology.

1. Gene Therapy: This revolutionary approach aims to correct genetic defects that cause endocrine disorders. By introducing healthy genes into the body, gene therapy can potentially provide a lifelong cure for certain conditions like congenital adrenal hyperplasia and growth hormone deficiency. Students will explore the principles behind gene therapy, its challenges, and the promising results observed in preclinical and clinical trials.

2. Stem Cell Therapy: Stem cells have the remarkable ability to differentiate into various cell types, making them a promising avenue for regenerative medicine. In the realm of endocrinology, stem cell therapy holds potential for treating conditions such as type 1 diabetes and hypoparathyroidism. This section will introduce students to the fascinating world of stem cells and their role in reshaping the future of pediatric endocrinology.

3. Artificial Pancreas: For children with type 1 diabetes, managing blood glucose levels can be a constant challenge. The development of artificial pancreas systems, which combine continuous glucose monitoring and automated insulin delivery, has revolutionized diabetes care. Students

will learn about the components of an artificial pancreas, its benefits, and the ongoing research to optimize its performance.

4. Precision Medicine: As our understanding of individual genetic variations grows, the concept of precision medicine becomes increasingly relevant. This approach involves tailoring treatment plans to a patient's unique genetic makeup, ensuring personalized and effective care. Students will explore the potential applications of precision medicine in endocrinology, including hormone replacement therapy and targeted cancer treatments.

5. Telemedicine: In a world where access to specialized healthcare is not always readily available, telemedicine provides a promising solution. This section will introduce students to the concept of telemedicine and its applications in pediatric endocrinology. From remote consultations to real-time monitoring, telemedicine can bridge the gap between patients and endocrinologists, improving access to care and enhancing patient outcomes.

By familiarizing themselves with these emerging therapies and technologies, students will be well-equipped to navigate the ever-evolving landscape of pediatric endocrinology. As future endocrinologists, they will have the opportunity to contribute to further advancements and positively impact the lives of countless children and adolescents with endocrine disorders.

Future Directions in Pediatric Endocrinology

As students in the field of endocrinology, it is vital to stay updated on the latest advancements and emerging trends in pediatric endocrinology. The field is constantly evolving, and new directions are being explored to provide better care and treatment options for children with endocrine disorders. In this subchapter, we will discuss some of the future directions in pediatric endocrinology that will shape the way we understand and manage these conditions.

One of the exciting areas of research in pediatric endocrinology is the use of genetic testing and personalized medicine. With advancements in genetic technologies, we can now identify specific gene mutations that contribute to endocrine disorders. This knowledge allows for more accurate diagnoses and tailored treatment plans. Additionally, gene therapy holds promise for correcting genetic defects and potentially curing certain endocrine disorders in the future.

Another future direction in pediatric endocrinology is the exploration of novel therapies. Traditional treatments such as hormone replacement therapy have been effective, but researchers are now investigating alternative approaches. For example, stem cell therapy shows promise in regenerating damaged or malfunctioning endocrine organs. This could revolutionize the treatment of conditions like type 1 diabetes or growth hormone deficiency.

Advancements in technology will also play a crucial role in the future of pediatric endocrinology. Wearable devices and continuous glucose monitoring systems are already improving the management of diabetes in children. As technology continues to evolve, we can expect more innovative tools to aid in the diagnosis, monitoring, and treatment of various endocrine disorders.

Prevention and early intervention will continue to be key focuses in pediatric endocrinology. As our understanding of risk factors improves, strategies for preventing endocrine disorders can be developed. Early screening and intervention programs will ensure that children receive timely treatment, minimizing the long-term impact of these conditions.

Lastly, interdisciplinary collaboration will shape the future of pediatric endocrinology. Researchers, clinicians, and allied healthcare professionals from various fields will work together to address the complex nature of endocrine disorders. This collaboration will lead to a more comprehensive and holistic approach to care, improving outcomes for children with endocrine conditions.

In conclusion, the future of pediatric endocrinology is promising and full of exciting possibilities. Genetic testing, personalized medicine, novel therapies, advancements in technology, prevention, and early intervention, as well as interdisciplinary collaboration, will shape the field in the years to come. As students, it is essential to stay informed and engaged with these future directions to contribute to the progress of pediatric endocrinology and provide the best care for our young patients.

Chapter 8: Case Studies and Clinical Scenarios

Case Study 1: Growth Hormone Deficiency

Introduction:
Welcome to the first case study in our book, "The Growing Years: A Student's Journey into Pediatric Endocrinology." In this chapter, we will explore a fascinating condition known as Growth Hormone Deficiency (GHD). This case study will provide students with a comprehensive understanding of GHD, its causes, symptoms, diagnosis, and treatment options.

Understanding Growth Hormone Deficiency:
Growth Hormone Deficiency is a condition that occurs when the body does not produce enough growth hormone, which is responsible for stimulating growth, development, and overall body composition. It primarily affects children but can persist into adulthood if left untreated. This condition can have significant effects on a child's physical and emotional well-being, making it essential for students studying endocrinology to understand its nuances.

Case Study:
Meet Sarah, a ten-year-old girl who has been experiencing slower growth compared to her peers. Sarah's parents are concerned about her height and have sought medical advice. After undergoing a series of tests, it is revealed that Sarah has Growth Hormone Deficiency. This case study will follow Sarah's journey, from her initial symptoms to the diagnosis and treatment plan developed by her endocrinologist.

Causes and Symptoms:
In this section, we will delve into the various causes of GHD, including genetic factors, birth complications, brain tumors, and infections. We will explore the symptoms associated with GHD, such as short stature, delayed puberty, low energy levels, and increased body fat. By understanding the causes and symptoms, students will gain insight into the complexity of diagnosing GHD.

Diagnosis and Treatment:
The diagnosis of GHD involves a combination of physical examinations, growth charts, blood tests, and imaging techniques. This section will explain the diagnostic procedures in detail, allowing students to comprehend the process thoroughly. Additionally, we will explore the various treatment options available, such as growth hormone injections, lifestyle modifications, and psychological support. Students will gain knowledge about the potential benefits and side effects of treatment, ensuring a holistic understanding of patient care.

Conclusion:
This case study on Growth Hormone Deficiency provides students with a comprehensive overview of the condition, its causes, symptoms, diagnosis, and treatment. It allows students to develop a deep understanding of endocrinology, particularly in relation to pediatric patients. By exploring Sarah's journey, students will gain insight into the challenges faced by patients with Growth Hormone Deficiency, fostering empathy and shaping their future practice as healthcare professionals in the field of endocrinology.

Case Study 2: Type 1 Diabetes Mellitus

Introduction:

Welcome to Case Study 2 in our book, "The Growing Years: A Student's Journey into Pediatric Endocrinology." In this chapter, we will delve into the intricacies of Type 1 Diabetes Mellitus, focusing on its diagnosis, management, and the impact it has on the lives of children and adolescents. As aspiring endocrinologists, it is crucial to understand this condition and develop the knowledge and skills necessary to provide optimal care to our patients.

Understanding Type 1 Diabetes Mellitus:

Type 1 Diabetes Mellitus, also known as insulin-dependent diabetes, is a chronic autoimmune condition that affects children and adolescents. It occurs when the immune system mistakenly attacks and destroys the insulin-producing cells in the pancreas, leading to a deficiency of insulin. Insulin is vital for regulating blood sugar levels, and its absence results in elevated blood glucose levels, leading to various complications.

Diagnosis and Management:

Diagnosing Type 1 Diabetes Mellitus involves assessing the patient's symptoms, medical history, and conducting blood tests to measure blood glucose and detect the presence of specific autoantibodies. Once diagnosed, the management of this condition revolves around maintaining optimal blood glucose levels through a combination of insulin therapy, regular monitoring of blood sugar levels, a balanced diet, and regular physical activity.

Impact on the Lives of Children and Adolescents:

Living with Type 1 Diabetes Mellitus can be challenging for children and adolescents. It affects their daily routine, requiring constant monitoring of blood glucose levels, administering insulin injections or using insulin pumps, and adhering to a strict meal plan. Moreover, they may face social and emotional challenges, such as feeling different from their peers or experiencing fears of hypoglycemia or diabetic complications.

As future endocrinologists, it is crucial to provide comprehensive care to our patients. This includes not only managing their medical needs but also addressing their psychosocial well-being. By understanding the unique challenges faced by children and adolescents with Type 1 Diabetes Mellitus, we can offer them the support and resources they need to live fulfilling lives.

Conclusion:

In this chapter, we have explored the intricacies of Type 1 Diabetes Mellitus. From its diagnosis to its impact on the lives of children and adolescents, we have gained valuable insights into this chronic condition. As students interested in the field of endocrinology, it is vital to develop a deep understanding of Type 1 Diabetes Mellitus, as it will enable us to provide the highest quality of care to our patients.

Case Study 3: Congenital Adrenal Hyperplasia

Congenital Adrenal Hyperplasia (CAH) is a rare genetic disorder that affects the adrenal glands, which are responsible for producing essential hormones in the body. This case study aims to shed light on the diagnosis, management, and long-term implications of CAH, providing students with a deeper understanding of this condition within the field of endocrinology.

Diagnosing CAH can be challenging due to its wide range of symptoms and variations in severity. However, early detection is crucial to prevent life-threatening adrenal crises and ensure proper management. This case study follows the journey of Sarah, a 7-year-old girl who presented with ambiguous genitalia, a common sign of CAH in females.

Sarah underwent a series of diagnostic tests, including hormone level assessments and genetic testing, which confirmed a diagnosis of CAH. This discovery led to a comprehensive treatment plan involving hormone replacement therapy, which aims to restore the balance of hormones in the body.

The book then delves into the complexities of managing CAH, such as the importance of regular check-ups, hormonal adjustments, and the potential side effects of long-term steroid use. It highlights the collaborative effort between pediatric endocrinologists, geneticists, and other healthcare professionals to optimize Sarah's growth, development, and overall well-being.

Furthermore, the case study explores the emotional and psychological impact of living with CAH. It addresses the challenges faced by Sarah and her family, including the need for education and support networks to cope with the unique circumstances of this condition. The book emphasizes the importance of promoting awareness, acceptance, and inclusivity for individuals with CAH.

Finally, the case study discusses the long-term implications of CAH. It highlights the potential impact on fertility, bone health, and the need for lifelong monitoring. It also touches upon the advancements in research and treatment options that offer hope for individuals with CAH to lead fulfilling lives.

In conclusion, "Case Study 3: Congenital Adrenal Hyperplasia" provides an in-depth exploration of this complex condition within the field of endocrinology. It offers valuable insights into the diagnosis, management, and long-term implications of CAH through the journey of Sarah, a young girl living with this condition. This subchapter aims to educate students about the challenges and advancements in the field of pediatric endocrinology, fostering a deeper understanding and empathy towards individuals affected by CAH.

Chapter 9: Career Opportunities in Pediatric Endocrinology

Becoming a Pediatric Endocrinologist: Education and Training

If you are a student interested in the fascinating field of endocrinology and have a passion for working with children, then a career as a pediatric endocrinologist might be the perfect fit for you. This subchapter will guide you through the education and training required to become a successful pediatric endocrinologist.

Education is the foundation for any medical career, and becoming a pediatric endocrinologist is no exception. Aspiring students must first complete a bachelor's degree in a related field such as biology, chemistry, or biochemistry. This undergraduate education provides a strong scientific background necessary for the advanced medical studies ahead.

After obtaining a bachelor's degree, the next step is to gain admission to medical school. This highly competitive process involves taking the Medical College Admission Test (MCAT) and submitting applications to various medical schools. Once accepted, students embark on a four-year medical program, where they learn the fundamentals of medicine and gain clinical experience through rotations in different specialties.

Upon graduation from medical school, aspiring pediatric endocrinologists must complete a three-year residency program in pediatrics. During this time, they work closely with experienced physicians in various pediatric subspecialties, including endocrinology. This residency provides the necessary knowledge and skills to diagnose and manage a wide range of pediatric conditions.

Following the completion of a pediatrics residency, individuals interested in specializing in pediatric endocrinology must pursue a fellowship in this subspecialty. Pediatric endocrinology fellowships typically last three years and focus on in-depth training in the diagnosis and treatment of hormonal disorders in children. Fellows have the opportunity to work with experts in the field, conduct research, and gain hands-on experience in managing complex cases.

Throughout their education and training, students interested in endocrinology should actively seek opportunities to engage in research projects related to pediatric endocrinology. This could involve participating in clinical trials or conducting laboratory-based research. Engaging in research not only expands knowledge but also demonstrates dedication and passion for the field.

Ultimately, a career in pediatric endocrinology requires a lifelong commitment to learning and staying current with the latest advancements in the field. Pursuing this path will allow you to make a significant impact on the lives of children, helping them overcome hormonal imbalances and achieve a healthy and fulfilling life.

In conclusion, becoming a pediatric endocrinologist requires a solid educational foundation, including a bachelor's degree, medical school, a pediatrics residency, and a pediatric endocrinology fellowship. It is a challenging yet rewarding journey that enables you to specialize in the diagnosis and treatment of hormonal disorders in children. With dedication and perseverance, you can embark on this fulfilling career and become a vital member of the endocrinology community.

Other Professions in Pediatric Endocrinology

While doctors play a critical role in the field of pediatric endocrinology, there are several other professions that contribute to the care of children with endocrine disorders. These professionals work alongside physicians and collaborate to provide comprehensive and holistic care to their patients. In this subchapter, we will explore some of these other professions in pediatric endocrinology.

One important profession in pediatric endocrinology is that of the pediatric endocrine nurse. These nurses specialize in caring for children with endocrine disorders and play a vital role in the management and education of both patients and their families. They assist in performing diagnostic tests, administering medications, and providing support and guidance to families during the treatment process. Pediatric endocrine nurses ensure that patients receive the necessary care and are involved in their overall well-being.

Another crucial profession in this field is the pediatric endocrine dietitian. These specialized dietitians work closely with patients and their families to develop tailored dietary plans that address specific endocrine disorders. They provide guidance on proper nutrition, help manage weight-related issues, and offer dietary recommendations to optimize the overall health of children with endocrine conditions. By working closely with the medical team, pediatric endocrine dietitians contribute significantly to the overall treatment plan.

Psychologists also play a vital role in the field of pediatric endocrinology. Children with endocrine disorders often face unique psychological challenges due to the impact of their condition on their physical appearance, growth, and development. Pediatric endocrine psychologists provide counseling and support to help patients and their families navigate these challenges. They assist in coping with the emotional aspects of living with an endocrine disorder and help develop strategies to manage any psychological difficulties that may arise.

In addition to these professions, there are also social workers, genetic counselors, and research scientists who contribute to the field of pediatric endocrinology. Each of these professionals brings unique expertise and perspectives to the care and treatment of children with endocrine disorders.

As students interested in endocrinology, it is important to recognize the multidisciplinary nature of pediatric endocrinology and the collaboration that occurs between various professions. By understanding the roles and contributions of these professionals, we can develop a more comprehensive understanding of the field and work together to provide the best possible care for our future patients.

Volunteer and Internship Opportunities

As students interested in the field of pediatric endocrinology, it is crucial to actively seek out opportunities that allow us to gain hands-on experience and contribute to the field. One of the best ways to do this is by exploring volunteer and internship opportunities. These experiences not only provide valuable insights into the world of endocrinology but also offer a chance to make a difference in the lives of young patients.

Volunteering in a pediatric endocrinology setting can be a transformative experience. By dedicating your time and skills, you have the opportunity to witness the challenges and triumphs of patients struggling with endocrine disorders. Whether it is assisting with administrative tasks, organizing educational events, or providing emotional support to patients and their families, volunteering allows you to develop a deeper understanding of the impact of endocrine disorders on children's lives.

Internships, on the other hand, provide a more structured and immersive experience. Many hospitals and research institutions offer internship programs specifically designed for students interested in endocrinology. These programs typically provide a unique opportunity to shadow healthcare professionals, participate in clinical research, or even assist in patient care under supervision. The hands-on experience gained during internships can be invaluable in shaping your future career path and understanding the complexities of pediatric endocrinology.

Moreover, volunteering and interning in the field of endocrinology also allows you to network with professionals and build relationships that can open doors to future opportunities. By immersing yourself in the field, you can connect with mentors who can guide you in your educational and career endeavors. These connections can provide recommendations, offer advice, or even lead to research or job opportunities in the future.

Lastly, volunteering and interning in pediatric endocrinology not only benefits your personal and professional development but also contributes to the advancement of the field. By actively participating in research projects or clinical trials, you have the chance to contribute to medical advancements in the field of endocrinology. Your efforts could potentially lead to breakthroughs in the treatment and management of endocrine disorders, positively impacting the lives of countless children.

In conclusion, as students interested in pediatric endocrinology, it is crucial to seek volunteer and internship opportunities. These experiences offer a chance to gain valuable insights, contribute to the field, and make a difference in the lives of young patients. By actively engaging in these opportunities, you can enhance your understanding of endocrine disorders, build a network of professionals, and potentially contribute to medical advancements in the field. Embrace these opportunities, immerse yourself in the world of pediatric endocrinology, and take the first step towards a fulfilling career in this specialized field.

Chapter 10: Conclusion and Reflections on the Journey

Personal Reflections on the Study of Pediatric Endocrinology

As a student delving into the fascinating field of pediatric endocrinology, my journey has been filled with awe-inspiring moments and invaluable learning experiences. This subchapter aims to provide personal reflections on this captivating subject, specifically tailored for students with a keen interest in endocrinology.

Pediatric endocrinology focuses on the study of hormonal disorders in children, ranging from growth and puberty to diabetes and thyroid disorders. It is a field that requires a deep understanding of the intricate workings of the endocrine system and its impact on a child's overall development.

One of the most striking aspects of studying pediatric endocrinology is witnessing the profound impact that hormonal imbalances can have on a child's life. It is both humbling and inspiring to witness the transformative power of medical interventions in restoring a child's health and quality of life.

Moreover, the multidisciplinary nature of pediatric endocrinology has further enriched my learning experience. Collaborating with experts from various fields such as genetics, psychology, and nutrition has broadened my perspective and taught me the importance of a holistic approach to patient care.

The study of pediatric endocrinology also presents unique challenges. Understanding complex hormonal pathways and interpreting diagnostic tests can be daunting, but the sense of accomplishment that comes with unraveling a diagnostic puzzle is immensely rewarding. It requires dedication, perseverance, and a genuine passion for understanding the intricacies of the endocrine system.

Additionally, interacting with young patients and their families has been an enlightening experience. Building trust and rapport with children requires patience and empathy, and witnessing their resilience is a constant reminder of the importance of our work as future pediatric endocrinologists.

As students, it is essential to actively engage in research and stay updated with the latest advancements in the field. Pediatric endocrinology is a rapidly evolving specialty, with new treatment modalities and diagnostic techniques continuously emerging. Embracing a lifelong learning mindset is crucial to providing the best care for our future patients.

In conclusion, the study of pediatric endocrinology is a captivating and rewarding journey. It offers students a unique opportunity to understand the impact of hormonal disorders on a child's development, collaborate with experts from various disciplines, and make a lasting difference in the lives of young patients. Embrace the challenges, stay curious, and never underestimate the transformative power of knowledge in the field of pediatric endocrinology.

Future Perspectives and the Importance of Continuous Learning

As students venturing into the field of endocrinology, it is crucial to understand the future perspectives and the importance of continuous learning. The world of endocrinology is constantly evolving, and it is necessary for students to stay updated with the latest advancements and discoveries in this ever-evolving field.

The future of endocrinology holds immense potential for growth and innovation. With the rapid advancements in technology and research, we can expect to witness groundbreaking discoveries and revolutionary treatments for endocrine disorders. As students, it is important to be aware of these future perspectives and embrace them wholeheartedly.

Continuous learning is the key to success in the field of endocrinology. The field is vast and encompasses various aspects of the endocrine system, hormone regulation, and the treatment of endocrine disorders. To excel in this field, students must be committed to lifelong learning and intellectual growth. This involves staying updated with the latest research, attending conferences and seminars, and engaging in discussions with fellow students and professionals.

Continuous learning ensures that students are equipped with the knowledge and skills necessary to provide the best possible care for their patients. It allows us to stay at the forefront of medical advancements, enabling us to employ the most effective treatments and interventions for endocrine disorders. Furthermore, it fosters critical thinking and problem-solving skills, which are essential in diagnosing and managing complex endocrine conditions.

In addition to staying informed about the latest research and advancements, students must also cultivate a deep understanding of the importance of empathy and patient-centered care. Endocrine disorders often have a profound impact on patients' lives, and it is our responsibility to provide compassionate care and support. By continuously learning about the emotional and psychological aspects of endocrine disorders, students can develop a holistic approach to patient care.

In conclusion, the future of endocrinology holds immense potential for growth and innovation. As students, it is crucial to understand the importance of continuous learning to stay updated with the latest advancements in the field. Continuous learning not only equips us with the necessary knowledge and skills but also fosters empathy and patient-centered care. By embracing lifelong learning, we can contribute to the advancements in endocrinology and provide the best possible care for our patients.

9 798886 904890